YOUR KNOWLEDGE HAS VALUE

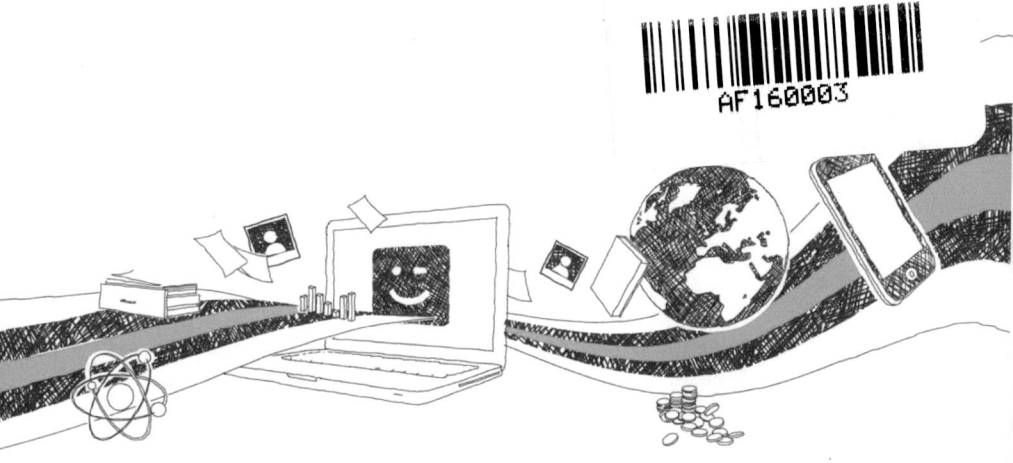

- We will publish your bachelor's and master's thesis, essays and papers

- Your own eBook and book - sold worldwide in all relevant shops

- Earn money with each sale

Upload your text at www.GRIN.com and publish for free

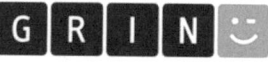

Bibliographic information published by the German National Library:

The German National Library lists this publication in the National Bibliography;
detailed bibliographic data are available on the Internet at http://dnb.dnb.de .

This book is copyright material and must not be copied, reproduced, transferred,
distributed, leased, licensed or publicly performed or used in any way except as
specifically permitted in writing by the publishers, as allowed under the terms and
conditions under which it was purchased or as strictly permitted by applicable
copyright law. Any unauthorized distribution or use of this text may be a direct
infringement of the author s and publisher s rights and those responsible may be
liable in law accordingly.

Imprint:

Copyright © 2018 GRIN Verlag
Print and binding: Books on Demand GmbH, Norderstedt Germany
ISBN: 9783668624535

This book at GRIN:

https://www.grin.com/document/388405

Patrick Kimuyu

Epilepsy Management. An Overview

GRIN Verlag

GRIN - Your knowledge has value

Since its foundation in 1998, GRIN has specialized in publishing academic texts by students, college teachers and other academics as e-book and printed book. The website www.grin.com is an ideal platform for presenting term papers, final papers, scientific essays, dissertations and specialist books.

Visit us on the internet:

http://www.grin.com/

http://www.facebook.com/grincom

http://www.twitter.com/grin_com

Epilepsy Management

Name: Patrick Kimuyu

Abstract 2
Introduction 3
Pathophysiology of Epilepsy 4
Partial Seizures 5
Generalized Seizures 5
First Aid Care During and After a Seizure 6
Drug Therapy 7
Principles of Anticonvulsant Therapy 7
Monotherapy Medications 7
Clonazepam 8
Lamotrigine 8
Gabapentin 8
Phenytoin 8
Sodium Valproate 9
Phenobarbital 9
Oxcarbazepine 9
Major Adverse Affects of Medications 9
Therapeutic Index of Anti-Epileptic Drugs 10
Recent Changes in Medical Care in Australia 10
Conclusion 10
References 12

Abstract

The principal aim of this report is to develop advanced understanding of the status of epilepsy, especially regarding its etiology, pathophysiology and treatment approaches. Therefore, I carried out an extensive research on epilepsy to gather the most relevant information on the disorder. In this research, I understood the definition of epilepsy and its history.

Epilepsy is defined as a brain disorder which occurs when neurons convey abnormal signals owing to interruptions in the process of generating electrochemical impulses. In practice, epilepsy is characterized by seizures in which neurons fire signals repeatedly.

Epilepsy does not have a universally acceptable cause, but there are some factors which are believed to contribute to the onset of the condition. Epidemiological studies reveal that epilepsy is associated to genetic factors, head trauma, infectious diseases, prenatal injury and some brain conditions. On the other hand, the pathophysiology of epilepsy involves two principal physiological mechanisms: ictogenesis and epileptogenesis. During ictogenesis, neuronal networks develop hyperexcitability, and this accounts for the signs and symptoms presented as seizures.

In practice, medical treatment for epilepsy involves a monotherapy in which a single drug is chosen to be administered to the patient based on the type of seizure observed. There are seven different pharmacological agents which are used for monotherapy. Some of the most common drugs used in the monotherapy are clonazepam, lamotrigine, gabapentin, phenytoin, sodium valproate, phenobarbital and oxcarbazepine. These drugs have diverse beneficial effects on different patients, and their dosages and modes of administration are also different. In addition, the indications and mechanisms of the drugs are different.

Currently, there are different types of seizures which are classified in accordance to the degree of consciousness, and drug therapy aims at eliminating the neuronal activity experienced during seizures.

This information enabled me to conclude that epilepsy is a significant brain disorder that requires attention by physicians and families.

Introduction

Epilepsy is defined as a brain disorder which occurs when neurons convey abnormal signals owing to interruptions in the process of generating electrochemical impulses. Ordinarily, neurons operate in a highly coordinated order to produce human feelings, thoughts and actions (Aicardi, Engel & Pedley, 2008). This neuronal activity is impaired in epileptic conditions in which strange behavior, sensations and emotions occur leading to muscle spasms, convulsions or even loss of consciousness.

In practice, epilepsy is characterized by seizures in which neurons fire signals repeatedly. It is reported that during a seizure, the neural system can produce more than 500 signals within a second, and this attributable to the abnormal activity of the nerve clusters in the brain.

Historically, epilepsy is known as the oldest mental illness to be identified by man. It dates back to 400 B.C when Hippocrates described it as a brain disorder. Currently, epilepsy has become an enormous challenge to the global public healthcare because it is not curable. This implies that, the management of epilepsy poses challenge to physicians although surgery techniques and medicines help in controlling seizures in 80 percent of epileptic patients. It is estimated that 2.5 million individuals in the US have been diagnosed with epilepsy (Goldenberg, 2010). However, experiencing a single seizure does not necessarily suggest epilepsy. This is why a comprehensive diagnosis is required in determining epilepsy and the different forms of seizures, in order to adopt the most appropriate treatment option. Therefore, this report will provide a comprehensive overview on epilepsy.

Etiology of Epilepsy

Epilepsy does not have a universally acceptable cause, but there are some factors which are believed to contribute to the onset of the condition. Epidemiological studies reveal that epilepsy is associated to genetic factors, head trauma, infectious diseases, prenatal injury and some brain conditions (Goldenberg, 2010).

Epilepsy has been found to run with families, and this suggests that some genes are responsible for the condition. Currently, about 500 genes have been identified to be involved in epileptic seizures. These genes have been found to influence an individual's response to environmental conditions. It is believed that some genes make some people more sensitive to some environmental stimuli which trigger seizures (Aicardi, Engel & Pedley, 2008).

On the other hand, brain conditions such as stroke and brain tumors can cause epilepsy because they cause brain damage. For instance, stroke and Alzheimer's have been identified as the leading cause of epilepsy, especially in old adults (Goldenberg, 2010). Head trauma has also been found to be a significant cause of epilepsy. In most cases, people with traumatic injuries resulting from car accidents and other injuries present with epilepsy. On the other hand, brain damage during the embryonic development of the fetus cause epilepsy more or less the same way as it occurs in cerebral palsy.

Infectious diseases and developmental disorders are also considered as significant causes of epilepsy. Some infectious diseases, especially those which cause brain damage such as meningitis, viral encephalitis and AIDS cause epilepsy. On the other hand, developmental disorders such as neurofibromatosis and autism are believed to play significant roles in the onset of epilepsy.

Pathophysiology of Epilepsy

The pathophysiology of epilepsy explains why some signs and symptoms are observed in epileptic patients. However, it is worth distinguishing the pathophysiology of epilepsy from seizures which are usually caused by the synchronous, excessive or abnormal neuronal activity in the patient's brain. Ordinarily, epileptic seizures are manifested by sensory auras, convulsive movements and altered awareness. Therefore, the pathophysiology of epilepsy explains the mechanisms involved in the initiation of epileptic seizures and the development of the patient's seizure-prone brain (Eisai, 2012).

The pathogenesis of epilepsy involves two principal physiologic mechanisms: ictogenesis and epileptogenesis. Ictogenesis is associated with hyperexcitation in the neural system. This excitation is believed to originate from different molecular sources including individual neurons, neuronal networks and the neuronal environment (Eisai, 2012). It is believed that functional, structural and physiologic changes in the postsynaptic membrane of neurons cause excessive excitation, and this causes seizures.

The spread of seizures and the effect of synaptic and nonsynaptic mechanisms play a significant role in epileptogenesis. During epileptogenesis, thalamocortical networks, synaptic, nonsynaptic and astrocytes play significant roles in the development of hypersynchronicity leading to ictal-interictal transition (Blumenfeld, 2003).

Types of Epileptic Seizures

Epileptic seizures are some of the most prevalent pediatric neurologic disorders among children, especially in children aged below three years. However, seizures occur in the first 16 years of the child's development and growth but, their frequency decreases with older age. Friedman and Sharieff (2006) state "seizures are the most common pediatric neurologic disorders, with 4% to 10% of children suffering at least one seizure in the first 16 years of life" (p. 257).

There are different forms of epileptic seizures which are grouped into two broad groups: partial and generalized seizures. In reality, these two types of seizures differ in the level of consciousness.

Partial Seizures

Partial seizures are usually localized to a specific area of the brain. The most prevalent types of partial seizures are simple partial seizures and complex partial seizures. In simple partial seizures, patients do not experience loss of consciousness or awareness (Goldenberg, 2010). On the other hand, complex partial seizures involve loss of consciousness.

Generalized Seizures

Generalized seizures are different from partial seizures in that, they begin all over the brain, and this is why they are described as generalized. Some of the most common generalized seizures include tonic-clonic seizures, myoclonic seizures, atonic seizures, absence seizures, and tonic seizures (Goldenberg, 2010).

Generalized tonic-clonic seizures, also referred to as grand mal seizures are among the group of generalized seizures, which causes considerable alteration of the child's level of consciousness. Grand mal seizures are known to be the most prevalent of all generalized seizures (Friedman & Sharieff, 2006).

Ordinarily, generalized tonic-clonic seizures are not localized to one side of the brain as it is the case with other forms of seizures. These seizures occur among children, usually in five distinct phases although the most conspicuous phases are the clonic and the postictal phases. The first phase involves the contraction of the child's body and the limbs, followed by the extension period in which the body straightens. The third phase is characterized with tremor, in which the child experiences rhythmic shaking and, the third phase, which is referred to as the clonic period, involves contraction and relaxation of the body muscles, characterized with continuous twitching of the limb and eye muscles. The postictal period is usually characterized with body aches, fatigue, severe headache and vision impairment. In general, generalized tonic-clonic seizures are believed to have a sudden onset but, they do not cause sensory or motor aura.

Absence seizures occur without warning signs, and they are rare. These seizures last for less that fifteen seconds and they are characterized by motionless stare (Goldenberg, 2010). It is reported that patients experiencing absence seizures regain alertness after the cessation of the seizure.

Myoclonic seizures are caused by abnormal neuronal activity in the brain stem in which muscle tone is increased. They are characterized by muscle jerking. Patients with myoclonic seizures experience changes in muscle tone. This type of seizures is related to atonic seizures, and they originate from the same brain location. In atonic seizures, muscles tend to go limp and the patient may crumble to the ground owing to the dramatic decrease of muscle tone (Goldenberg, 2010).

Another type of generalized seizures is clonic seizures in which muscles stiffen leading to the arching of the back and rolling back of the eyes. Other muscles which are affected by tonic seizures are the chest, legs and arm muscles. These seizures are fatal because the tightening of the chest muscles may result into breathlessness, and this explains why the patient's face and lips appear bluish.

First Aid Care During and After a Seizure

People experiencing seizures require appropriate first aid to prevent devastating health outcomes such as injuries, and even death, especially when seizures occur while the patient is in water. The first step to undertake in providing first aid to someone who is experiencing convulsions is to ensure the place is safe. The surrounding should be safe so, any objects should be moved away from the patient. However, it is worth noting that attempts to move the patient is not advisable; instead, objects such as furniture and other objects that can cause injury to the patient should be taken away from the patient. It is also worth reassuring other people; ensure that they are calm (CDC, 2011).

The second step involves easing the patient to the ground and placing a supportive material such as a folded jacket under the head. Thereafter, ensure the patient breath properly by loosening any cloth around the neck such as ties, and eyeglasses should also be removed. The last step is timing the start of a seizure. In situations where the seizure persists for more than 5 minutes, seeking for emergency medical attention is recommended (CDC, 2011).

After the seizure, the patient is supposed to be put into the recovery position. Turning the patient to lie by the sides enhances breathing. It is also crucial to ensure that the airway is not blocked, either by food or any other substance. The patient should also be checked for injuries or recurrence of another seizure soon after the first one ends.

Drug Therapy

Anti-epileptic drug therapy has always been the mainstay for the management of epileptic seizures. It is reported that 80% of people who present with epileptic seizures show recovery after drug therapy, although surgery contributes to the successful management of the condition. Ideally, drug therapy involves four principal goals since the disorder is not curable. This means that some patients who experience seizures throughout their lifetime are put on regular drug administration, and this may cause some health consequences such as drug toxicity.

The first goal of drug therapy is to reduce the frequency of seizures. This is necessary for patients who experience frequent seizure episodes. In some cases, drug therapy eliminates the seizures. The second goal of anti-epileptic drug therapy is to prevent adverse effects, especially in long-term treatment with AEDs. It also helps patients in restoring or maintaining their usual vocational and psychological activities. Fourthly, drug therapy for epilepsy aims at maintaining the patient's normal lifestyle.

Principles of Anticonvulsant Therapy

On the other hand, the initiation of anti-epileptic drug therapy requires the consideration of some factors. Despite the controversy whether therapy should be considered for a single seizure, the decision to initiate the drug therapy is supposed to be based on the consequences of recurrent seizures, informed analysis which reveals the possibility of seizure recurrence, and the adverse and beneficial effects of the anti-epileptic drugs chosen for the treatment regime.

In most cases, the monitoring of seizures during AED therapy helps in determining whether the patient is responding appropriately to the treatment. It also enables physicians to identify any adverse effects caused by the chosen pharmacological agent.

Monotherapy Medications

In practice, medical treatment for epilepsy involves a monotherapy in which a single drug is chosen to be administered to the patient based on the type of seizure observed. There are seven different pharmacological agents which are used for monotherapy. Some of the most common drugs used in the monotherapy are clonazepam, lamotrigine, gabapentin, phenytoin, sodium valproate, phenobarbital and oxcarbazepine.These drugs have diverse beneficial effects on different patients, and their dosages and modes of administration are also different. In addition, the indications and mechanisms of the drugs are different.

Clonazepam

Clonazepam is useful for patients with myoclonic seizures or Lennox-Gastaut syndrome which is commonly referred to as petit mal variant. It is also useful in treating absence seizures in patients who do not show appreciable response to succinimides. Evidence shows that 30% of epileptic patients on clonazepam record significant loss of anti-seizure activity within 3 months of monotherapy. Therefore, re-adjustment is considered as a reliable approach for re-establishing efficacy.

In children, daily dosage of clonazepam ranges from 0.01 to 0.03 mg/kg, and it should not exceed the daily dosage of 0.05 mg/kg which is divided into three doses. On the other hand, adults should be administered with clonazepam on a daily dosage of 1.5 mg, in which the maximum daily dosage is set at 20mg (Malow & Sato, 2005).

Lamotrigine

Lamotrigine is used for the treatment of partial and generalized tonic-clonic seizures; especially in patients aged over two years. This agent diminishes neuronal activity by inactivating voltage-sensitive Na^+ channels. Lamotrigine is administered to patients at a dosage of 25 mg/day, especially within the first two weeks, and then dosage is increased to 50 mg/day (Goldenberg, 2010).

Gabapentin

Gabapentin is used for the treatment of partial seizures in patients without secondary generalization of seizures. This drug is administered orally in three doses a day which do not exceed 1,800 mg/day. In practice, the gabapentin is initiated at a dose of 300 mg/day, and then the dose is increased up to 1,800 mg/day. In patients aged five years and above, gabapentin is administered in three doses at a range of 25-35 mg/kg, daily, although initiation doses range from 10-15 mg/kg.

Phenytoin

Phenytoin is used for the control of complex partial seizures and generalized tonic-clonic seizures. It also prevents the occurrence of seizures during neurosurgery. This agent inhibits the spread of neuronal seizure activity by exerting its effects on the motor cortex. As such, it responds to hyperexcitability which is usually caused by excessive stimulation in the brain. Initiation of phenytoin involves 400 mg dosages. Thereafter, patients are administered with 300 mg dosages at two-hour intervals. In pediatric patients, 5 mg/kg per day is considered for initial administration, whereas the recommended maintenance dose is 4-8 mg/kg (Goldenberg, 2010).

Sodium Valproate

Sodium valproate is indicated for partial and generalized seizures. This agent acts by increasing the concentration of chemical transmitters such as GABA in the brain. However, its mechanism on how it exerts its anti-seizure activity has not yet been identified.

In monotherapy, valproate is initiated at a dosage of 10-15 mg/kg per day. Thereafter, the dose is increased by 1 mg/kg, in order to achieve its optimal clinical response. In most cases, plasma concentrations ranging from 50 to 100 mcg/mL are considered sufficient to attain optimal clinical response.

Phenobarbital

Phenobarbital is used for the treatment of seizures in neonates, although it is effective for treating partial and generalized tonic-clonic seizures in adults. This agent acts on the postsynaptic membrane and reduces the rate of neurotransmitter release by regulating calcium channels.

In practice, Phenobarbital concentration of 10-25 mcg/mL is believed to achieve anti-seizure activity in epileptic patients. This plasma concentration is achieved by administering the agent at doses of 15 to 20 mg/kg. In AED therapy, Phenobarbital is given in three daily doses ranging from 50 to 100 mg (Goldenberg, 2010).

Oxcarbazepine

Oxcarbapezine is indicated for patients with partial seizures. It is one of the most reliable drugs for monotherapy and adjunctive therapy. This agent stabilizes hyperexcitability of synaptic membranes by blocking voltage-sensitive Na^+ channels. The drug is administered orally at a dosage of 1,200 mg/day, especially during the initiation of monotherapy. However, a dose of 2,400 mg/day is recommended for patients switching monotherapy from other agents (Goldenberg, 2010).

Major Adverse Affects of Medications

In most cases, antiepileptic drugs are associated with adverse effects. This is so because some medications are continued for long-term. Clonazepam is associated with alopecia, anemia, amnesia, and ankle edema. It also causes anorexia, aphonia, chest congestion and choreiform movements. On the other hand, gabapentin causes ataxia, cramps and vaginal bleeding in females (Goldenberg, 2010).

Lamotrigine is associated with bipolar disorder, ataxia and blood dyscrasias. It also causes drug contraindication with oral contraceptives. On the other hand, Phenobarbital causes agitation, anxiety, apnea and bradycardia. It also causes depression in epileptic patients. Oxcarbapezine causes anaphylactic reactions, diplopia and fatigue. Finally, phenytoin is associated with ataxia, asterixis and arthralgias. It also causes hepatoxicity which may result into liver failure or damage, and headache disorder (Goldenberg, 2010).

Therapeutic Index of Anti-Epileptic Drugs

Therapeutic index is defined as the plasma concentration level at which a therapeutic drug achieves optimal clinical response. In reality, different anti-epileptic drugs exhibit varied therapeutic indices. For instance, Phenytoin has a therapeutic index of 10-20 mcg/mL, whereas Phenobarbital therapeutic index is 10-30 mcg/mL. On the other hand, Carbamazepine and Sodium Valproate have therapeutic indices of 5-12 mcg/mL and 50-100 mcg/mL, respectively (Greco et al., 2011).

Recent Changes in Medical Care in Australia

Over the years, treatment for epilepsy has been changing owing to the results obtained in research studies on the condition. In Australia, the management of epilepsy is governed by the recent management guidelines which were released in 2013. These guidelines state the clinical measures to be observed in managing epilepsy. For initial support, physicians are supposed to monitor oxygen saturation, whereas acute management of epilepsy should ensure supportive care of up to 10 minutes. It is also recommended that patients with seizures for more than 5 minutes be given benzodiazepine and dextrose IV infusion (Government of South Australia, 2013).

Conclusion

Conclusively, epilepsy is one of the most prevalent brain disorders. This disorder is characterized by seizures, and it etiology is associated to genetic factors, head trauma, infections and other mental disorders such as Alzheimer's and meningitis.

The pathophysiology of epilepsy involves two principal physiological mechanisms: ictogenesis and epileptogenesis. During ictogenesis, neuronal networks develop hyperexcitability, and this accounts for the signs and symptoms presented as seizures. On the other hand, epileptogenesis occurs when changes in the nervous system transforms normal brain morphology to seizure-prone brain.

Ordinarily, there are different types of seizures which are classified in accordance to the degree of consciousness, and drug therapy aims at eliminating the neuronal activity experienced during seizures. However, the treatment and management of epilepsy in Australia has been changing in which new guidelines are introduced to address different challenges, and improving the treatment outcomes in patients. Therefore, it is apparent that epilepsy requires significant attention from healthcare professionals, as well as the public.

References

Aicardi, J., Engel, J. & Pedley, T. (2008). *Epilepsy: A Comprehensive Textbook, Volume 3.* Sydney, Australia: Lippincott Williams & Wilkins.

Blumenfeld, H. (2003). From Molecules to Networks: Cortical/Subcortical Interactions in the Pathophysiology of Idiopathic Generalized Epilepsy. *Epilepsia,* 44(2):7-15.

CDC (2011). *First Aid for Seizures.* Retrieved from http://www.cdc.gov/epilepsy/basics/first_aid.htm

Eisia (2012). *Pathophysiology of Epilepsy.* Retrieved from http://www.focusonepilepsy.com/pdfs/pathophys.pdf

Friedman, M. & Sharieff, G. (2006). Seizures in Children. *Pediatr Clin N Am,* 53, 257 – 277. doi:10.1016/j.pcl.2005.09.010.

Goldenberg, M. (2010). Overview of Drugs Used For Epilepsy and Seizures: Etiology, Diagnosis, and Treatment. *Pharmacy & Therapeutics,* 35(7): 392–415. Retrieved from http://www.ncbi.nlm.nih.gov/pmc/articles/PMC2912003/

Government of South Australia (2013). *SA Paediatric Clinical Guidelines: Management of seizures in children.* Retrieved from https://www.google.com/url?sa=t&rct=j&q=&esrc=s&source=web&cd=10&cad=rja&uact=8&ved=0CHkQFjAJ&url=http%3A%2F%2Fwww.naml.com.au%2Fmedia-resources%2Fclinical-resources%3Fdownload%3D29%3Astatewide-paediatric-guidelines-final-draft-management-of-seizures&ei=y8qEU6bMK469uASJ2IC4DA&usg=AFQjCNGJBq41hdzSCY-XMEBL0Uc6a3xFtg&sig2=Micx4gitO7jKN37uBJohjA&bvm=bv.67720277,d.c2E

Greco, F. A. et al. (2011). *Therapeutic Drug Levels.* Retrieved from http://www.nlm.nih.gov/medlineplus/ency/article/003430.htm

Malow, B. & Sato, S. (2005). *Benzodiazepines: Clonazepam.* New York, NY: Raven Press.

YOUR KNOWLEDGE HAS VALUE

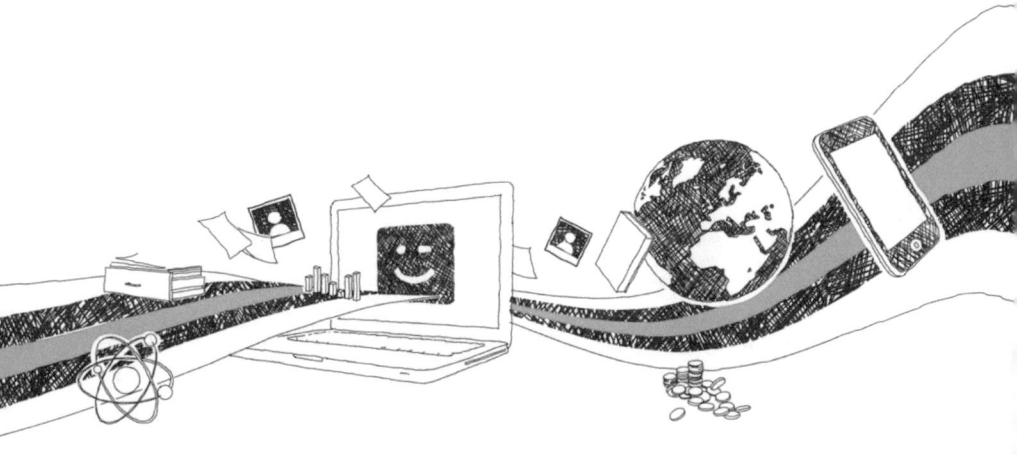

- We will publish your bachelor's and master's thesis, essays and papers

- Your own eBook and book -
  sold worldwide in all relevant shops

- Earn money with each sale

Upload your text at www.GRIN.com
and publish for free

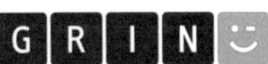